A book that might save you someday

My dad has cancer

By

M.

A BOOK THAT MIGHT SAVE YOU SOMEDAY (MY DAD HAS CANCER)

First edition. February 16, 2025.

ISBN: 979-8230174073

Written by M..

Table of Contents

Preface

Cancer. It's a word that changes lives in an instant. When my dad was diagnosed with **non-small cell lung cancer (NSCLC) stage 3B, mucoepidermoid carcinoma grade 2 variant**, our world turned upside down.

Doctors told us the options were limited, the prognosis was grim, and the road ahead would be anything but easy. The pulmonologist told us that this cancer is rare and they do not have an established chemotherapy treatment for it. Radiation is deemed too risky as the location of the tumour is near the aorta. Also, surgery carries a huge risk for the same reason. It was estimated that the tumour could double in size within 90 to 180 days from the day of diagnosis.

On top of everything, my dad was also diagnosed with lymphangitic carcinomatosis (LC)—a condition where cancer cells spread through the lymphatic system of the lungs, causing inflammation and obstruction. This meant that his cancer wasn't just a single mass; it had infiltrated the tiny lymphatic channels in his lungs, making breathing more difficult over time. Studies have reported that approximately 50% of patients succumb within three months of symptom onset, and only about 15% survive beyond six months. But instead of surrendering to fear, we decided to fight in our own way.

This book isn't a miracle cure. It's not a replacement for medical advice. It's simply the story of what we did, what we learned, and what we wish we had known sooner. If you or someone you love is facing cancer, I hope this **$12 book** offers you something valuable—whether it's **hope, a new perspective, or even just a small piece of information that could make a difference.**

Throughout this journey, we explored **alternative treatments, diet changes, and unconventional strategies** alongside medical opinions. Every step taught us something that might help others walking the same difficult path. Before we go deeper into this journey, let's look at something important—the CT scans taken 81 days apart. When we first received his diagnosis, we were told the tumour could double in size within 90 to 180 days, a terrifying prospect. But when we compared the two scans, something unexpected happened. It hadn't progressed. Some areas even showed signs of improvement—a rare moment of relief in an otherwise overwhelming battle. Despite everything, his condition remained stable. In the world of cancer, stability is a victory.

I wrote this book because **if even one sentence in here helps you or your loved one, then it was worth it.**

This is our story. Maybe, just maybe, it might save you someday.

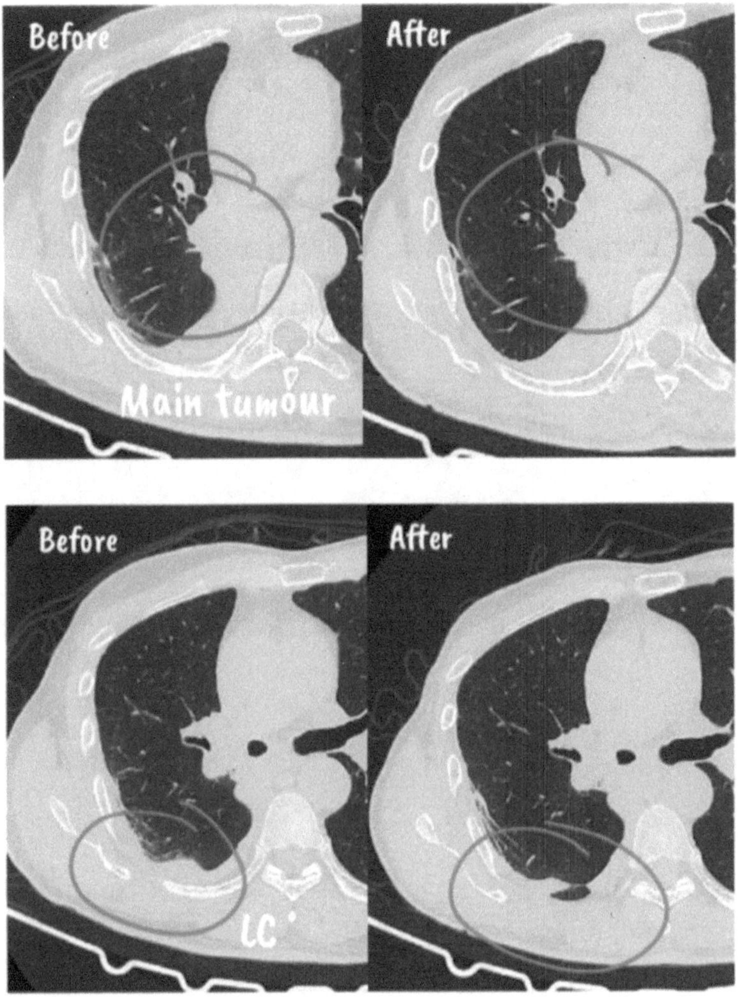
Before
After
Main tumour
Before
After
LC

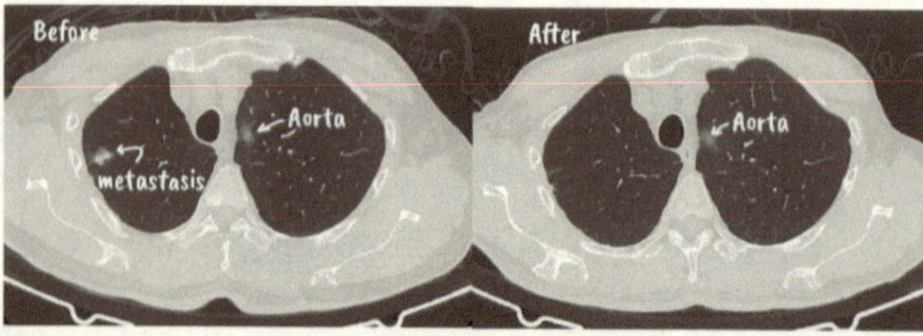
Before
After
Aorta
metastasis
Aorta

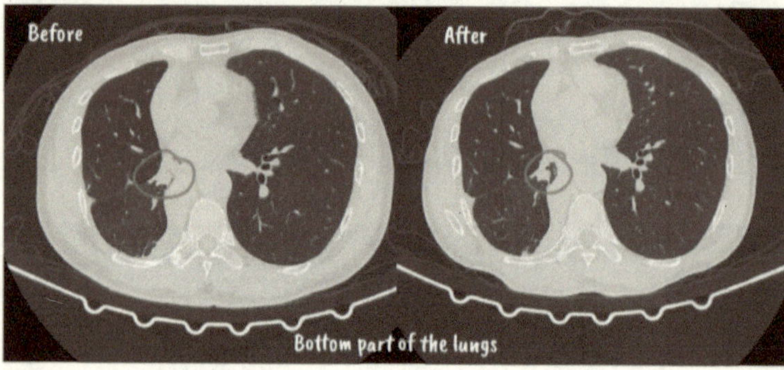
Before
After
Bottom part of the lungs

Chapter 1: A Life of Hardship, Sacrifice, and Unfairness

Dad **grew up struggling from a young age**, taking on responsibilities far beyond his years. At just **11 years old**, he was already **digging his own well, riding a bicycle to the market to sell ornamental fish, and running from officials because he didn't have a license**—all to support his family of six after his father abandoned them.

Despite his immense efforts, life kept throwing obstacles at him. He built a **fish-selling business** with blood, sweat, and tears, only to be **betrayed and kicked out at 40** because his **mother favoured his idle younger brother**. Even before losing the business, he was barely making **RM300–400 a month**, while his mother **hoarded the profits**. Still, he **remained loyal and hardworking**, thinking it was all for the family.

Even after starting over from scratch, he remained **honest and kind** in his work, always **giving the best advice** and using **high-quality treatments** for his customers' fish. But **rich and entitled customers constantly took advantage of his kindness**—demanding discounts despite driving luxury cars, talking behind his back, and assuming he was earning a huge profit when, in reality, his margin was **barely 20-40%**. Some months, his income was **zero**, and he even had to take **overdraft loans to keep the family afloat**. Because of this **financial instability**, he couldn't afford to send me and my sister to university. I had to study hard to secure a place in public university. I pursued a degree in Aquaculture, and my thesis focused on using traditional Chinese medicine to kill bacteria that cause secondary infections in fish. It was a success and the herb holds the key in saving fishes without the use of antibiotics.

Now, at **68 years old**, after a lifetime of **hard work and sacrifice**, he has **0 savings, 0 retirement funds, and now, stage 3B rare mucoepidermoid carcinoma (MEC) lung cancer**. A cancer **so rare that there is no proper chemotherapy or immunotherapy available**. He never smoked or drank, yet life still dealt him this cruel hand.

After enduring a **childhood of abandonment, a lifetime of exploitation, and financial struggles**, he now faces the **biggest battle of his life**.

Chapter 2: The Day Everything Changed

My dad had been coughing for almost four months. At first, it was mild, just a little irritation here and there, nothing out of the ordinary. But as time went on, it lingered, and it grew more persistent. Then, one day, there was blood—just a little, but enough to make me worry. I told him to check it out. "It's probably nothing," he said, waving off my concern. He had always been like that—tough, resilient, the kind of man who wouldn't let a simple cough slow him down. He had worked through far worse in his life. Cancer? That wasn't even a thought in his mind.

Maybe he would have continued ignoring it if not for my sister's invitation. She wanted him to come to Australia for eight months to spend time with her and help take care of her son. He was excited—after all, it wasn't often that he got the chance to take a break, to be with family without the weight of work on his shoulders. But there was a catch. To get his visa approved, he needed a medical check-up. Just a routine process, nothing to be concerned about. Or so we thought.

As part of the medical requirements, he went for a chest X-ray. That's when everything changed. The results came back showing something. A shadow. An abnormality in his lung. The doctor wasn't sure what it was, but it wasn't normal. We needed more tests. We were required to run TB test to test for tuberculosis and it was negative. The CT scan came next, giving us a clearer picture of what was inside his lungs. And then, the biopsy—the test that would confirm our worst fears. I remember waiting for the results, hoping for the best but bracing for the worst. When the diagnosis came back, it was cancer.

The report was in his hands. The first biopsy report. We hadn't even seen the doctor yet, but the words were already there, printed in black and white. I looked at him, waiting for a reaction. Then I saw it—the defeated look on his face. It broke me. My dad had always been strong. He had endured so much in life without ever showing weakness. But at that moment, I saw something in him I had never seen before—fear. The realization that this wasn't just a bad cough. That this was something bigger. Something life-changing. He didn't say a word. Neither did I. We both just stared at the report, as if not reading it out loud would somehow change its meaning. For the first time in my life, my dad looked vulnerable. And I wasn't ready for that.

He underwent a PET scan to determine if the cancer had spread further. Then an MRI to check for brain metastases. Every test, every scan, every appointment was a step deeper into a reality we never thought we'd face. All in all, it was non-small cell lung cancer (NSCLC), stage 3B, mucoepidermoid carcinoma, grade 2. A rare form of lung cancer. The kind where no standard chemotherapy treatment existed. Radiation is not possible because of the tumour location being too near to the aorta. Surgery is too risky for the same reason, and 25 percent chance of dying on the surgery table, another 25 percent within 30 days after the surgery, another 25 percent within 90 days. And just like that, everything changed. The man who had survived so much now had to face something even more unforgiving.

In the days that followed, we found ourselves drowning in a sea of medical terms, survival rates, and treatment options—most of which offered little hope. It felt like we were being pushed into a corner, with nowhere to go.

Then, one day, we came across an interview by DOAC with Dr. Thomas Seyfried.

For two hours, we sat there, watching, listening. His words made sense. He spoke about cancer in a way we had never heard before—not just as an unstoppable force but as something that could be starved, controlled, and fought in unconventional ways.

For the first time since we got the diagnosis, we felt hope. This wasn't just blind optimism—it was a new way of understanding the enemy. If we were going to fight this, we had to know what we were up against. So, we went deeper.

We started digging through research papers, watching more interviews, reading scientific journals. The more we learned, the more we realized that the standard path wasn't the only one. There were other approaches—ones that weren't widely accepted, but ones that offered possibilities.

If there was even the slightest chance to help my dad, we had to try.

Chapter 3: Understanding the Enemy

For most of my life, I believed that cancer was purely genetic. This was what I was taught in university genetics courses, and it was the prevailing narrative in modern medicine—cancer is caused by mutations in DNA, and once those mutations accumulate, the cell turns cancerous.

But when my dad was diagnosed, I started questioning everything. I came across a new perspective, one that shifted my entire understanding of cancer. It wasn't just about genetics. Cancer is a disease of the mitochondria.

The Experiment That Changed Everything

There was a study that challenged the genetic theory of cancer. In this experiment:

-A healthy nucleus was placed inside a cancer cell. The cell still behaved like a cancer cell.

-A cancerous nucleus was placed inside a healthy cell. The cell remained healthy.

If cancer were purely genetic, replacing the nucleus—the home of our DNA—should have "fixed" the cancerous cell. But it didn't. Instead, this experiment suggested that the true problem isn't in the nucleus, but in the mitochondria—the powerhouse of the cell.

Genetics and Cancer: A Misunderstood Link

Yes, there are cancer-driving genes, but they don't automatically turn a normal cell into cancer. They increase the likelihood of developing cancer, but whether or not cancer actually forms depends on whether those genes are activated. In fact, every single person has dormant cancer genes in their body. If these genes are never triggered, cancer never develops. This means that something else must be responsible for pushing a normal cell into a cancerous state.

How Cancer Grows and Spreads

When cancer first develops, it is often small enough to evade the immune system. It may start producing rogue cells that float around the body. White blood cells (WBCs) can usually detect and destroy these abnormal cells, but here's the terrifying part:

After millions of attempts, one cancer cell may survive long enough to latch onto another part of the body. This is how metastasis happens. However, not all metastasized cells survive. If a cancer cell ends up in an environment different from its origin, it may struggle to grow. But if it finds a similar environment—one that favours its survival—it thrives and spreads. That is why it very common to see metastases happen near the source first before it can be found in distant parts of the body.

Cancer's Survival Strategy: Hijacking Glucose and Glutamine and Creating a Shield

Cancer loves **glucose and glutamine**. It thrives on them. Unlike healthy cells, which can switch between different energy sources, cancer cells are heavily dependent on glucose for survival. Here's how they protect themselves:

Cancer consumes glucose and glutamine rapidly, using them as fuel to grow.

It releases succinic acid and lactic acid as by-products.

These acids create a highly acidic environment around the tumour.

This prevents white blood cells from attacking, because immune cells cannot survive in an overly acidic environment.

Essentially, cancer builds a chemical shield around itself, making it nearly untouchable by the body's natural defences.

And the acid can kill nearby healthy cell too. This breaks down those healthy cells around them into building blocks and the cancer can now use those building blocks for themselves.

Glutamine is a non-essential amino acid that the body produces naturally and is also obtained from dietary protein. It plays a crucial role in cell growth, immune function, and nitrogen transport. Under normal conditions, it supports muscle repair, gut health, and brain function.

Why does cancer use glutamine?

Glutamine feeds the mitochondria, allowing cancer to generate ATP (energy) even in the absence of glucose.

It helps cancer cells build nucleotides (DNA & RNA), fatty acids, and proteins, essential for rapid growth.

Glutamine is involved in antioxidant production, which protects cancer cells from oxidative stress and chemotherapy-induced cell death.

Where does glutamine come from?

Dietary sources: High-protein foods like meat, fish, dairy, eggs, soy, legumes, and nuts.

Internal production: The body naturally synthesizes glutamine from other amino acids in the muscles and liver.

This explains why simply cutting out sugar isn't enough—cancer can adapt and use other fuels like glutamine. But I am not saying you should stop taking proteins. We need proteins for our immune system too. If you stop taking proteins, your health will definitely deteriorate in many ways.

Cancer May Be Able to Camouflage

Cancer hides from immune surveillance by expressing immune checkpoint molecules (like PD-L1), tricking white blood cells into ignoring them.

This is why immune checkpoint inhibitors (a type of immunotherapy) have been developed to "unmask" cancer cells. However, it is an expensive treatment. My dad's cancer type is rare, so there is no established immunotherapy for him.

A New Way of Looking at Cancer

This new understanding completely changed my perspective. Instead of seeing cancer as a fixed genetic fate, I started seeing it as a metabolic disease—one that could be influenced, starved, or slowed down by controlling its energy sources.

Chapter 4: Our Strategy

Once we understood how cancer worked, we realized that traditional treatments weren't our only option. My dad's cancer was rare, and there was no established immunotherapy for him. The standard approach—chemotherapy and radiation—was either ineffective or too risky due to the location of his tumour.

So, we had to think differently.

Our strategy revolved around four key principles:

1. **Starving the Cancer** – Cutting off its fuel sources.
2. **Boosting the Immune System** – Strengthening the body's natural defences.
3. **Correcting Deficiencies** – Addressing weaknesses that could make him more vulnerable.
4. **Utilising Repurposed Drugs** - Drugs that have shown potential in cancer treatment.

1. Starving the Cancer

We knew that cancer relies heavily on glucose and glutamine to survive. If we could disrupt its energy supply, we could slow its growth.

The Role of Diet: A Metabolic Approach

Since cancer is metabolically inflexible, meaning it struggles to use fats or ketones as fuel, we focused on:

A strict low-carb, high-fat ketogenic diet to reduce glucose availability.

Time-restricted eating & fasting to lower insulin and force cancer cells into a vulnerable state.

Targeting glutamine metabolism (since cancer can use both glucose and glutamine).

Cancer cells thrive on sugar, but healthy cells can adapt to burning fat and ketones—this gave us an edge in cutting off cancer's primary fuel.

Foods such as potatoes, rice, bread, carrots, and anything that can eventually be broken down into glucose are either restricted or severely minimized. We rely on Google and ChatGPT to check whether certain foods contain carbohydrates. Some people said cancer patients should try juicing or eat more fruits. Well, if the fruit is sweet, you have to avoid it. It has sucrose which eventually breaks down into glucose and fructose. Some cancer patients may not survive even if they try juicing, as the vegetables they choose might contain too many carbohydrates like carrots. Hence, we have to search online to make sure that what he eats contains minimal carbohydrates. Carbohydrates contents should be lower than 20g or 30g.

Our body can use ketones for energy when glucose is scarce. I, too, switched to a zero-carb diet for an entire month to understand the physiological changes the body experiences when eliminating carbohydrates. Despite the dietary shift, I was still able to work as usual and continued jogging three times a week. The first few days left me feeling a bit lightheaded, but after that, I felt more energetic than ever.

Intermittent fasting has become a daily norm for my dad. He also practises a 24-hour fast once a week, commonly known as one meal a day (OMAD). Occasionally, his 24-hour fast extends to 36 hours, depending on his endurance. His weight is monitored daily to track any signs of muscle loss, malnutrition, or unexpected weight fluctuations that could indicate underlying issues. It helps adjust protein and fat intake if necessary to maintain a stable condition. Without carbohydrates, it is very hard for him to gain weight due to the absence of glucagon which is crucial component to form adipose tissue.

Remember the main fuels for cancer? Other than glucose, glutamine. To limit glutamine for the cancer, he limits animal proteins because they contain relatively high levels of glutamine, which could potentially fuel cancer growth. All proteins (animal or plant) have glutamine because glutamine is a naturally occurring amino acid found in most protein-rich foods. We cannot eliminate glutamine completely because of its importance. Hence, exercise and always opt for plant protein are the answers. If you want to take egg, only consume the yolk as the white contains a lot of glutamines. Another useful tip is to use any AI to help you figure out which food has high glutamine.

Muscle Consumption of Glutamine

Skeletal muscles are the largest glutamine reservoir in the body.

When you exercise, muscles use up glutamine for recovery, reducing the amount available in the bloodstream.

This means less glutamine for cancer cells to use as fuel.

Shifting Glutamine to the Immune System

Exercise stimulates immune cells, especially lymphocytes and macrophages, which also use glutamine as an energy source.

This diverts glutamine away from cancer cells, making it harder for tumours to thrive.

Increased Glucose & Fat Oxidation

Exercise promotes the body's shift toward burning glucose and fat for energy, reducing cancer's metabolic advantage.

By improving insulin sensitivity, it helps prevent excess glucose from being easily available for tumour growth.

Regulation of Tumour Microenvironment

Moderate exercise can help reduce inflammation and oxidative stress, both of which cancer exploits to grow.

Some studies suggest that exercise lowers lactate accumulation, which prevents tumours from creating their acidic shield against immune attacks.

Best Types of Exercise for Cancer Patients

-Aerobic Exercise (e.g., walking, jogging, cycling) – Helps burn excess glucose and shift metabolism.

-Strength Training (e.g., bodyweight exercises, light resistance training) – Depletes muscle glutamine stores, making less available for cancer.

-High-Intensity Interval Training (HIIT) – Short bursts of intense activity can rapidly deplete energy stores, making it harder for cancer to adapt.

We did some search online on how much protein does he need according to his weight. Some days he gets 100% of what he needs, some days he gets 70% of what he needs.

To maintain his energy levels, my dad's diet is predominantly high in fat. He consumes three tablespoons of extra virgin olive oil with every meal. Occasionally, he swaps extra virgin olive oil for MCT oil, as different oils serve different purposes.

Extra virgin olive oil (EVOO) is rich in monounsaturated fats and polyphenols, which have anti-inflammatory and cardioprotective effects.

MCT oil (medium-chain triglycerides) is rapidly absorbed and converted into ketones, making it a quick energy source.

Given the high-fat intake, I was initially concerned about its effect on his blood pressure, especially since his systolic pressure had consistently been over 140 mmHg prior to this dietary change. However, with this diet, his pressure has now dropped to below 120 mmHg, a remarkable improvement.

2. Boosting the Immune System

If cancer was hiding from the immune system, then our next move was to strengthen his immune response to help his body fight back.

Vitamin D and T-Cell Activation

My dad was diagnosed with osteopenia 10 years ago. At the time, we didn't think much of it. But now, we see it as a possible sign of long-term vitamin D deficiency—and that deficiency could have weakened his immune system.

Vitamin D is essential for activating T cells, the body's immune soldiers. Without enough vitamin D, T cells remain dormant, unable to detect and attack threats like cancer.

This made supplementing vitamin D3 a priority.

Dosage: 4000IU of Vitamin D and 200mcg of K2 daily.

*Taking K2 prevents overdosing Vitamin D complications.

Other Immune-Boosting Strategies

Sulforaphane (Found in broccoli sprouts)

20-40mg daily

-Supports detoxification by activating phase II liver enzymes.

-Has anti-cancer properties by inhibiting tumour growth and inducing apoptosis (cell death) in cancer cells.

-Reduces oxidative stress and chronic inflammation, both of which fuel cancer progression.

Cordyceps (Medicinal mushroom)

450mg/500mg daily

-Enhances immune system function by stimulating natural killer (NK) cells.

-Improves oxygen uptake and energy levels, which may help counteract cancer-related fatigue.

-Contains polysaccharides with anti-tumour effects, potentially slowing cancer growth.

Astragalus + Scutellaria Baicalensis (Infusion)

8g of Astragalus dried root and 6g of Scutellaria Baicalensis dried root.

-Astragalus: Boosts immune function.

-Scutellaria Baicalensis (Chinese Skullcap): Contains baicalein, which has anti-cancer, anti-inflammatory, and antioxidant properties.

-This combination is often used in Traditional Chinese Medicine (TCM) for immune support and cancer prevention.

Clinacanthus Nutans (Infusion) (Sabah Snake Grass)

-Traditionally used in Southeast Asia as a cancer treatment.

-Known for its anti-inflammatory, anti-viral, and anti-tumour properties.

-Some studies suggest it may inhibit cancer cell proliferation and reduce oxidative stress.

White Tea

-Rich in catechins, which have strong anti-cancer effects by preventing tumour cell growth.

-Contains powerful antioxidants that help neutralize free radicals.

-Has a milder caffeine content than green or black tea, making it gentler on the body.

Curcumin + Black Pepper (Turmeric extract & Piperine)

-500mg daily

-Curcumin (from turmeric) is a potent anti-inflammatory and anti-cancer compound that can inhibit multiple cancer pathways.

-Black pepper (piperine) enhances curcumin absorption by up to 2,000%, making it far more effective.

-Curcumin has been shown to suppress tumour growth, block metastasis, and reduce chemotherapy side effects.

…n

… wake up his immune system and remove any …at might have been suppressing it.

…prepare herbal infusions?

…nsure maximum retention of bioactive compounds, follow …ese steps when preparing herbal infusions:

1. Boil the water – Bring water to a boil.
2. Let it cool slightly – Allow the temperature to drop to 90-93°C before proceeding.
3. Steep the herbs – Pour the hot (not boiling) water over the herbs in a pot.
4. Let it infuse – Allow the herbs to steep until the infusion cools down.
5. Serve and enjoy – Drink warm or at room temperature.

Important Note:

Avoid using excessively high temperatures as they can denature too many bioactive compounds, reducing the infusion's effectiveness.

I did this for my thesis and the results were promising. So, yeah, infusion works!

3. Correcting Deficiencies & Strengthening His Body

Cancer patients often suffer from micronutrient d
making their bodies weaker and more vulnerable. We r
restore balance and ensure his body had everything it ne
function optimally.

Vitamin D3 & K2 – To help with both immunity and
health.

Omega-3 fatty acids – To reduce inflammation.

B vitamins & electrolytes – To maintain energy levels and
cellular repair.

By addressing deficiencies, we weren't just fighting cancer—we were improving his overall quality of life so he could withstand the battle ahead.

4. Utilising Repurposed Drugs

In addition to diet, fasting, and supplements, we also explored repurposed drugs that have shown potential in cancer treatment. Among them, we used:

1. Mebendazole (MBZ) – The Anti-Parasitic with Anti-Cancer Potential

Originally used to treat parasitic worm infections, mebendazole has gained attention for its anti-cancer effects.

It works by disrupting microtubules, which are essential for cancer cell division and tumor growth.

Studies suggest it can:

I. Inhibit cancer cell proliferation
II. Block angiogenesis (the formation of new blood vessels that feed tumors)
III. Trigger apoptosis (programmed cell death in cancer cells)

Unlike traditional chemotherapy, mebendazole selectively targets cancer cells while leaving healthy cells mostly unaffected.

Mebendazole (MBZ) Dosage

Standard Cancer Dose: 600 mg per day

Divided into: 200 mg thrice daily

With Food: Best taken with a fatty meal to enhance absorption.

Duration: 3 times daily for 3 days then rest for 4 days.

Safety: Generally well-tolerated, but long-term use should be monitored for liver function and blood counts.

Mechanism of Action in Cancer:

-Inhibits microtubule formation, preventing cancer cell division.

-Starves tumors by blocking glucose uptake.

-May act synergistically with other treatments like metformin or fenbendazole.

2. Ivermectin – More Than Just an Anti-Parasitic

Known for treating parasitic infections, ivermectin has been studied for its potential anti-cancer properties.

Some research indicates it can:

I. Disrupt cancer cell metabolism
II. Inhibit tumor growth by affecting key signaling pathways
III. Enhance immune response against cancer cells

Ivermectin is also believed to work synergistically with other treatments, making it a promising addition to a broader cancer-fighting strategy.

Ivermectin Dosage

Standard Cancer Dose: 0.2 – 0.4 mg per kg of body weight per day

Example:

For a 70 kg (154 lbs) person, the dose would be 14 mg – 28 mg daily.

With Food: Best taken with a fatty meal for better absorption.

Duration: Taken daily at 12mg and occasionally 24mg straight for 3 days.

Safety: Well-tolerated, but can cause dizziness, nausea, or mild neurological effects in sensitive individuals.

Mechanism of Action in Cancer:

Disrupts cancer cell metabolism and weakens mitochondrial function.

Inhibits WNT/β-catenin signaling, which many cancers use for growth.

May enhance immune response against cancer cells.

We knew there were no guarantees. But if this approach could slow progression, improve his health, or even give him more time, then it was worth doing.

It is also important to give his body some break for consuming too much supplements and drugs. Only supplements that does not stress the liver can be continued such as vitamin D and cordyceps. Hence, he takes a break of 4-5 days after every 3 weeks of supplementing.

These drugs have shown potential anticancer effects through various mechanisms, primarily disrupting cellular processes critical for cancer cell survival and proliferation. Below is a breakdown of their hypothesized mechanisms:

Mechanism	Ivermectin	Mebendazole	Fenbendazole	Albendazole
Microtubule Disruption	No	Yes	Yes	Yes
Oxidative Stress	Yes	No	Yes	Yes
Apoptosis Induction	Yes	Yes	Yes	Yes
Angiogenesis Inhibition	No	Yes	No	Yes
Energy Starvation	Yes	No	Yes	Yes
Immune Modulation	Yes	No	No	Yes
WNT/β-catenin Inhibition	Yes	No	No	No

As of now, we are sticking to using ivermectin and mebendazole as they are more widely known and documented for human use.

Diets

Morning: Avocado, egg, olive oil, and curcumin + black pepper powder

Lunch: Some protein (plant proteins such as tofu, occasionally take fish protein), olive oil, a lot of green leafy or cruciferous vegetables, and curcumin + black pepper powder.

Dinner: Some protein (plant proteins), olive oil, a lot of green leafy or cruciferous vegetables, curcumin + black pepper powder, low carbohydrate cheese and butter.

1 Plant protein is often preferred over animal protein for cancer patients due to several important health, metabolic, and biochemical reasons that align with cancer management goals:

◈ 1. Lower Glutamine and Methionine Content

- Many tumours, especially aggressive ones, are "addicted" to glutamine and methionine, which are found in higher amounts in animal proteins (e.g., beef, chicken, fish).
- Plant proteins like tofu, lentils, and peas have lower levels of these amino acids, which may starve tumour cells or reduce their growth signals.

◈ 2. Anti-inflammatory Properties

- Plant-based foods are naturally rich in anti-inflammatory compounds such as:
    - Polyphenols (e.g., from green tea, berries)

  - Flavonoids (e.g., in soy, beans)
  - Fibre (feeds gut bacteria → produces butyrate → anti-inflammatory)
- In contrast, processed meats and red meats can increase inflammation, which fuels cancer progression.

◈ 3. Lower IGF-1 Stimulation

- Insulin-like Growth Factor 1 (IGF-1) is a hormone that promotes cell growth and division.
- High animal protein intake has been linked to elevated IGF-1, which can stimulate tumour growth.
- Plant proteins generally do not spike IGF-1 to the same degree, especially when from legumes, nuts, or seeds.

◈ 4. Fibre and Gut Microbiome Support

- Plant protein sources are often rich in fibre, which:
  - Promotes a healthy gut microbiome.
  - Enhances immune function.
  - Produces beneficial short-chain fatty acids that may protect against colorectal and other cancers.
- Animal proteins contain zero fibre.

◈ 5. Fewer Toxins and Carcinogens

- Cooking animal protein at high temperatures (grilling, frying) can produce heterocyclic amines (HCAs) and polycyclic aromatic hydrocarbons (PAHs) – both are carcinogens.

- Processed meats (bacon, sausages) also contain nitrates/nitrites, linked to colorectal cancer.
- Plant proteins don't form these carcinogens during cooking.

◈ 6. Alkaline vs. Acidic Load

- Animal proteins are acid-forming and may:
  - Disrupt body pH homeostasis.
  - Promote chronic low-grade inflammation.
- Most plant-based proteins are more alkaline-forming, which supports overall health and potentially better outcomes in cancer therapy.

◈ 7. Ethical and Sustainable Choices

- Although not directly health-related, many cancer patients adopt plant-based diets for environmental or ethical reasons, which can contribute to their sense of well-being and purpose—important in healing.

◈ Best Plant Protein Sources for Cancer Patients

Protein Source	Notes
Tofu / Tempeh	Complete protein, rich in isoflavones (anti-cancer in some studies)
Lentils/ Chickpeas	High in fibre, low in methionine, support gut health
Pumpkin seeds	High in zinc, magnesium, and protein
Pea protein isolate	Useful for shakes, low allergen risk
Hemp seeds	Complete protein, anti-inflammatory fats
Chia seeds	Omega-3s and fibre, good for smoothies
Edamame	Young soybeans, lower in glutamine than meat

2 Olive Oil vs. MCT Oil

- **If olive oil is not consumed, MCT oil is the substitute.**

Why Use Olive Oil?

- **Rich in monounsaturated fats & polyphenols** → **Anti-inflammatory & heart-protective**.
- **Supports mitochondrial function** → Helps reduce oxidative stress, which cancer thrives on.
- **Lowers blood pressure** → Important because your dad previously had high BP (~140 mmHg).

Why Substitute with MCT Oil?

- **Faster Ketone Production** → MCTs (Medium-Chain Triglycerides) bypass normal digestion and are quickly converted into ketones, providing an **immediate energy source** for healthy cells but **not cancer cells.**
- **Appetite Regulation** → MCTs may help counteract **cachexia** by improving caloric intake and satiety.
- **Easier Digestion** → Ideal when fat tolerance is lower or **when immediate energy is needed.**

When to Use MCT Instead of Olive Oil?

- **When extra energy is needed quickly** (before workouts or when feeling fatigued).
- **When fat digestion is compromised** (e.g., if digestion is sluggish, MCT is absorbed faster).

3 Small Amounts of Berries as Dessert

Why Berries?

- **Low Glycaemic Index (GI)** → Berries **don't cause a large blood sugar spike**, making them a **keto-friendly fruit.**
- **Rich in Antioxidants** → High in **polyphenols (ellagic acid, quercetin, anthocyanins)**, which may have **anti-cancer properties.**
- **Supports Brain & Heart Health** → Protects against oxidative stress and inflammation.

Why Only Occasionally?

- Even though they are **low-carb,** berries **still contain natural sugars**, so **excessive intake can disrupt ketosis.**
- **Maintaining strict glucose restriction** is crucial to limiting **cancer's primary energy source.**

Which Berries Are Best?

- **Raspberries, Blackberries, Strawberries → Lowest in sugar, highest in fibre and antioxidants.**

- **Avoid Grapes, Bananas, Apples** → Too high in **sugar and carbs.**

4 Low-Carb Yogurt & Nuts (Almonds/Macadamias) as Snacks

Why Low-Carb Yogurt?

- **Probiotic Benefits** → Supports **gut health and immune function.**
- **Protein Source** → Helps maintain **muscle mass without excessive glutamine intake.**
- **Lower Insulin Response** → Unlike regular yogurt, **low-carb versions** minimize **blood sugar spikes.**

Best Choice: Greek yogurt (full-fat, unsweetened, low-carb brands).

Why Almonds & Macadamia Nuts?

- **High in Healthy Fats** → Supports **ketosis and energy balance.**
- **Rich in Magnesium & Antioxidants** → Helps regulate **inflammation and mitochondrial function.**
- **Macadamia Nuts Are Best** → **Lowest in carbs**, highest in **monounsaturated fats.**

Why Not Cashews or Peanuts?

- **Cashews** → **Higher in carbs**, can disrupt ketosis.
- **Peanuts** → **Contain lectins**, which may trigger inflammation in some people.

5 Reading Nutrient Facts for All Products

Why Every Product Must Be Checked for Carbs?

- Hidden sugars & starches are **everywhere**, even in "healthy" foods.

- Many packaged foods **contain glucose, maltodextrin, or fillers** that can **feed cancer cells.**

- Strict carb control ensures **ketosis remains stable**, keeping cancer under metabolic pressure.

Key Ingredients to Watch Out For:

- **Sugar, Maltodextrin, Dextrose** → Spike blood sugar.

- **"Low-Fat" or "Fat-Free" Labels** → Usually means **added sugars.**

- **Vegetable Oils (Soybean, Corn, Canola, Sunflower)** → Promote **inflammation.**

Golden Rule:

Always choose whole, unprocessed foods whenever possible to ensure **full control over nutrient intake.**

Final Summary: The Logic Behind Every Choice

1 **Choose plant protein** over animal proteins most of the time.

2 **Olive oil and avocado are the preferred fat source**, but **MCT oil is used when fast energy is needed.**

3 **Berries are only consumed occasionally** to **avoid glucose spikes**, while still providing antioxidants.

4 **Low-carb yogurt and nuts** help maintain **gut health and satiety** without disrupting ketosis.

5 **Every food label is carefully checked** to ensure **no hidden carbs** interfere with the metabolic strategy.

Chapter 5: How Did Our Family Embrace the Uncertainty

Cancer doesn't just affect the patient—it shatters the entire family. When my dad was diagnosed, the weight of it crushed us all in different ways.

I cried until my left ear went deaf for a week. My sister cried so much that a blood vessel in her eye burst. My mom was just silent—too overwhelmed to even process what was happening.

It wasn't easy. I spent hours reading and reading. Searching for things that could help my dad and could be explained in science. Then came up with this strict regime for him.

How do you prepare for something like this? How do you keep going when the person you love is facing something so terrifying and unpredictable?

We didn't have the answers, but we knew one thing: we had to make every moment count.

Holding Onto Happiness Amidst the Pain

We decided to do everything we could to lighten the mood, to make sure my dad's days weren't filled with just doctor visits, medications, and medical research.

I took him and my mom on a vacation—something he never had the luxury of doing before. We visited places he couldn't afford in the past, places he once thought he would never see.

For a brief moment, cancer wasn't the centre of everything.

We laughed, took pictures, and ate meals together like any normal family would. It wasn't about running away from reality—it was about making new memories, despite reality.

The Little Things That Kept Us Going

Faith – My family turned to prayer, believing that if nothing else, faith would give us the strength to keep going.

Laughter – We made it a point to joke around, to remind ourselves that life wasn't over yet.

Sticking Together – We stopped taking each other for granted. Every day became more meaningful, every conversation more important.

New Experiences – Instead of focusing on what he might lose, we focused on what he could still do.

The fear never really left us. But we learned to live with it—not in despair, but with the determination to make every day count.

What This Taught Us

Cancer had stolen so much from us. But it also gave us clarity.

It reminded us that life is fragile, uncertain, and completely out of our control. But that doesn't mean we should spend it drowning in fear.

Instead, we chose to embrace the uncertainty—to cry when we needed to, but also to laugh, to love, and to live.

And that made all the difference.

Chapter 6: Results and What's Next

As you can see from the scans in the Preface, the results speak for themselves.

A metastasis in the upper lung has cleared.

Lymphangitic carcinomatosis (LC) appears to be improving.

The lower part of the lung seems to be shrinking.

The main tumour hasn't progressed significantly—despite the initial expectation that it would double in size within months.

By all medical expectations, it should have been worse. But it's not.

How He Feels Now

Beyond the scans, the biggest proof is how he feels.

Breathing has improved. The chronic cough that lingered for months is gone.

He tells me he feels like his lung volume has increased. I take it with a grain of salt, but the fact that he notices a difference means something.

His back pain is gone. He used to struggle with discomfort, but now, he can crouch without difficulty, something that was tough before.

He has increased his workout intensity. Compared to the first two months, he now does more intensive exercises to keep himself active.

The biggest concern? His weight.

He's skinnier now, technically underweight. Cancer, combined with keto and fasting, has stripped away some of his mass.

Cachexia (muscle loss) is always a worry. But with workouts and a controlled diet, I hope to counteract it.

What's Next?

We are not stopping here.

Continuing the current approach – The diet, fasting, supplements, repurposed drugs, and exercise will remain key.

Adjusting to counter weight loss – Finding ways to maintain muscle mass without feeding cancer.

Ongoing scans and monitoring – Watching closely to ensure stability or further improvements.

Exploring new metabolic strategies – Always learning, always adapting.

This journey isn't over. But for now, we've won some battles.

And that gives me hope.

Chapter 7: Literature Review

Can Anti-Parasitic Drugs Really Help Fight Cancer?

There's been a lot of buzz about repurposing anti-parasitic drugs for cancer treatment, and honestly, it's pretty fascinating. Some of these drugs, originally designed to kill parasites, have shown unexpected anti-cancer effects in lab studies and even some real-life cases. Let's break down what the research says about albendazole, mebendazole, ivermectin, and fenbendazole—without the complicated science talk.

Albendazole – The Parasite Killer That Attacks Cancer Too?

Albendazole is normally used to **kill parasitic worms**, but researchers found that it also **messes up cancer cells' ability to divide and grow**.

How it works:

- It **disrupts microtubules**, which are like highways inside cells. Without them, cancer cells can't divide properly.
- It **increases oxidative stress**, basically putting cancer cells under pressure until they break down.

What studies say:

- It has slowed down tumour growth in lab tests on **breast and liver cancer cells**.
- Some early reports suggest it might **help alongside**

chemotherapy, but there's not enough human trial data yet.

The catch?

- There aren't enough human studies to say it's a sure thing.
- Could cause **liver stress**, so long-term use needs careful monitoring.

Albendazole Induces Immunotherapy Response by Facilitating PD-L1 Degradation

These findings propose that albendazole could be repurposed to improve the effectiveness of existing cancer immunotherapies by targeting and degrading PD-L1 on tumor cells.:

https://jitc.bmj.com/content/10/5/e003819

Albendazole inhibits colon cancer progression and therapy resistance by targeting ubiquitin ligase RNF20

This study reveals that albendazole promotes antitumor immunity by inducing ubiquitin-mediated PD-L1 protein degradation, suggesting its potential to enhance immunotherapy responses.:

https://experts.nebraska.edu/en/publications/albendazole-inhibits-colon-cancer-progression-and-therapy-resista

Albendazole Exhibits Anti-Neoplastic Actions Against Gastric Cancer Cells

Findings suggest that albendazole can modulate the activation of STAT3 and STAT5 by pleiotropic mechanisms in gastric cancer cells, leading to apoptosis.:

https://www.mdpi.com/2227-9059/9/4/362

Mebendazole – The Dewormer That Disrupts Cancer's Growth

Mebendazole is another anti-worm drug that's being explored for **brain tumours (glioblastoma), lung cancer, and melanoma**.

How it works:

- **Stops cancer cells from dividing** by messing with their structural framework.
- **May help starve tumours** by blocking their ability to form new blood vessels.

What studies say:

- It has been tested against **glioblastoma (aggressive brain cancer)** and showed **some tumour reduction**.
- Some cancer patients using it off-label **have reported slower disease progression**.

The catch?

- Again, **not enough big clinical trials** to prove it works for everyone.

- Works best **when combined with other treatments**, not as a stand-alone cure.

Albendazole and Mebendazole as Anti-Parasitic and Anti-Cancer Agents: an Update

This provides a comprehensive review of the uses of **albendazole** and **mebendazole**, two broad-spectrum anthelmintic (anti-parasitic) medications.:

https://pmc.ncbi.nlm.nih.gov/articles/PMC8255490/

Mebendazole Treatment Disrupts the Transcriptional Activity of Hypoxia-Inducible Factors in Breast Cancer

This research demonstrates that mebendazole inhibits the transcriptional activity of hypoxia-inducible factors in breast cancer cell lines and mouse models, suggesting its potential as a cancer therapy.:

https://pmc.ncbi.nlm.nih.gov/articles/PMC9954103

Repurposing Drugs in Oncology (ReDO)—Mebendazole as an Anti-Cancer Agent

This article discusses the potential of mebendazole as an anti-cancer agent, highlighting its efficacy in preclinical models and case reports, particularly in adrenocortical cancer.:

https://ecancer.org/en/journal/article/443-repurposing-drugs-in-oncology-redo-mebendazole-as-an-anti-cancer-agent

Mebendazole Prevents Distant Organ Metastases in Part by Suppressing Tumour Platelet Aggregation

The study indicates that mebendazole has low toxicity and efficacy in multiple cancer models, including breast cancer, and may prevent metastases by suppressing tumour-induced platelet aggregation.:

https://breast-cancer-research.biomedcentral.com/articles/10.1186/s13058-022-01591-3

Emerging Perspectives on the Antiparasitic Mebendazole as a Repurposed Drug for the Treatment of Brain Cancers

This review explores mebendazole's potential as a treatment for brain tumours, discussing its efficacy both as monotherapy and in combination with standard treatments.:

https://www.mdpi.com/1422-0067/24/2/1334

Johns Hopkins Study: Anti-Parasitic Drug Slows Pancreatic Cancer in Mice

This study shows that mebendazole may slow pancreatic cancer progression in mice by collapsing cancer cells' structure and reducing inflammation.:

https://www.hopkinsmedicine.org/news/newsroom/news-releases/2021/08/johns-hopkins-study-anti-parasitic-drug-slows-pancreatic-cancer-in-mice

Ivermectin – More Than Just a Controversial Drug?

Yes, ivermectin—the same drug that stirred up controversy during the pandemic—is being studied for its **potential anti-cancer effects.**

How it works:

- It blocks **the WNT/β-catenin pathway**, which some aggressive cancers use to grow uncontrollably.
- It might **boost the immune system's ability to recognize and attack cancer cells.**

What studies say:

- Some lab studies show it **slows down tumour growth** in certain cancers, like **breast and colon cancer**.
- Some researchers believe it could **work alongside chemotherapy** to make treatment more effective.

The catch?

- Most research is **still in the early stages**—no solid proof yet that it works in real-life patients.
- A few case reports look promising, but **we need more trials** to confirm anything.

Ivermectin: A Multifaceted Drug With a Potential Beyond Anti-Parasitic Therapy

This comprehensive review discusses ivermectin's potential applications beyond its antiparasitic role, including its effects on various cancer cell lines. The study highlights how ivermectin may induce apoptosis (programmed cell death) and inhibit proliferation in cancers such as breast cancer and glioblastoma. However, the authors emphasize that most findings are from laboratory studies, and clinical trials are necessary to confirm efficacy in humans.

https://pmc.ncbi.nlm.nih.gov/articles/PMC11008553

Ivermectin Has New Application in Inhibiting Colorectal Cancer Cell Growth

This research explores ivermectin's effects on colorectal cancer cells, demonstrating that it can inhibit cell proliferation and induce apoptosis (cell death) in a dose-dependent manner. The study suggests that ivermectin may have potential as a therapeutic agent for colorectal cancer, though further research is needed.:

https://www.frontiersin.org/journals/pharmacology/articles/10.3389/fphar.2021.717529/full?utm_source=chatgpt.com

Ivermectin, a potential anticancer drug derived from an antiparasitic drug

This article explores the potential use of ivermectin, traditionally an antiparasitic medication, as an anticancer agent. The authors review various mechanisms by which ivermectin may inhibit cancer development and promote programmed cell death, suggesting its promise in cancer therapy. They also discuss prospects for its clinical application in treating neoplasms.:

https://pubmed.ncbi.nlm.nih.gov/32971268/

The multitargeted drug ivermectin: from an antiparasitic agent to a repositioned cancer drug

This review highlights that the antitumor activities of ivermectin observed in vitro and in vivo are achieved at concentrations attainable in humans, based on existing pharmacokinetic studies. This suggests the potential for repurposing ivermectin in cancer treatment, warranting further clinical trials to evaluate its efficacy and safety in oncology.:

https://pubmed.ncbi.nlm.nih.gov/29511601/

Fenbendazole – The "Joe Tippens Protocol" Drug

Fenbendazole is a **dog dewormer** that became famous when a cancer patient, **Joe Tippens**, claimed it helped him beat terminal lung cancer. That got people curious.

How it works:

- Like mebendazole, it **blocks microtubules**, stopping cancer cells from multiplying.
- It may also **cut off cancer's energy supply** by affecting glucose metabolism.

What studies say:

◈ Some lab studies show it **slows down certain cancer cells**, like colon and lung cancer.

◈ But so far, **no proper clinical trials** have confirmed its effectiveness in humans.

The catch?

- Most evidence comes from **personal stories**, not solid scientific studies.
- While it seems safe, it's **not officially approved for cancer treatment**, and doctors remain sceptical.

Oral Fenbendazole for Cancer Therapy in Humans and Animals

This comprehensive review discusses fenbendazole's anticancer activities, including its ability to inhibit glycolysis, reduce glucose uptake, induce oxidative stress, and promote apoptosis in cancer cells. The authors also address the drug's pharmacokinetics, bioavailability challenges, and potential strategies to enhance its therapeutic efficacy.:

https://ar.iiarjournals.org/content/44/9/3725

Anti-Cancer Effects of Fenbendazole on 5-Fluorouracil-Resistant Colorectal Cancer Cells

Investigating drug-resistant cancer models, this study reveals that fenbendazole induces apoptosis and cell cycle arrest in 5-fluorouracil-resistant colorectal cancer cells. The findings suggest that fenbendazole may serve as an alternative treatment for cancers that have developed resistance to conventional therapies.:

https://pmc.ncbi.nlm.nih.gov/articles/PMC9437363

Anti-Cancer Effect of Fenbendazole-Incorporated PLGA Nanoparticles in Chemo-resistant Ovarian Cancer

Addressing the challenge of fenbendazole's poor water solubility, this research explores the use of PLGA nanoparticles to enhance its delivery and efficacy. The study demonstrates that fenbendazole-loaded nanoparticles exhibit significant anticancer effects in chemo-resistant ovarian cancer models, suggesting a promising approach to improve therapeutic outcomes.:

https://doi.org/10.3802/jgo.2023.34.e58

Why the Ketogenic Diet Can Kill Cancer, According to Dr. Thomas Seyfried

Dr. **Thomas Seyfried**, a leading researcher in cancer metabolism, proposes that **cancer is primarily a metabolic disease, not just a genetic one**. His research suggests that cancer cells rely on **glucose (sugar) and glutamine** for survival and that **cutting off these fuel sources through a ketogenic diet can help slow or even kill cancer cells**.

Here's a breakdown of **why** the **ketogenic diet** may be effective against cancer, according to Dr. Seyfried's research:

1 Cancer Cells Are Metabolically Defective

Normal cells can switch between burning glucose (sugar) and ketones (fat) for energy.

Cancer cells, however, have defective mitochondria and struggle to use ketones for energy.

This means cancer cells are highly dependent on glucose and glutamine—without them, they struggle to survive.

Seyfried's Conclusion: If you cut off glucose and glutamine, cancer cells are starved, while normal cells adapt and thrive on ketones.

2 The Warburg Effect: Cancer Thrives on Glucose, Not Fat

Otto Warburg (a Nobel-winning scientist) discovered that cancer cells use a different method of energy production called "aerobic glycolysis" (Warburg Effect).

Even in the presence of oxygen, cancer cells prefer fermenting glucose rather than using mitochondria for efficient energy production.

Ketogenic diets drastically reduce glucose availability, forcing normal cells to switch to ketones while cancer cells struggle.

Seyfried's Conclusion: By starving cancer of glucose, you take away its primary fuel source, leading to tumour shrinkage.

3 Ketones Protect Healthy Cells, But Cancer Cells Can't Use Them

A ketogenic diet (high fat, very low carb) forces the body into ketosis, where it produces ketone bodies (β-hydroxybutyrate).

Healthy cells can efficiently use ketones for energy, but cancer cells cannot because of their damaged mitochondria.

This creates a metabolic environment where healthy cells survive, but cancer cells are weakened.

Seyfried's Conclusion: Ketones act as a metabolic shield, nourishing normal cells while leaving cancer cells to starve.

4 A Ketogenic Diet Reduces Insulin & IGF-1, Slowing Cancer Growth

High-carb diets stimulate insulin and IGF-1 (Insulin-like Growth Factor-1), which promote cancer cell growth and metastasis.

The ketogenic diet lowers insulin and IGF-1, reducing cancer growth signals.

Seyfried's Conclusion: Lower insulin and IGF-1 levels slow cancer progression and reduce tumour growth.

5 Fasting & Ketosis Activate Autophagy (Cancer Cell Self-Destruction)

Fasting and a ketogenic diet trigger autophagy, the body's natural process of clearing out damaged cells, including cancer cells.

Cancer cells struggle under these conditions, as they lack the flexibility to adapt to nutrient deprivation.

Seyfried's Conclusion: Intermittent fasting + ketosis puts pressure on cancer cells, making them more vulnerable to death.

6 Combining the Ketogenic Diet with Other Cancer Therapies (Press-Pulse Strategy)

Seyfried suggests a "Press-Pulse" strategy to maximize cancer cell death while minimizing harm to normal cells:

- Press = Constant glucose and glutamine restriction (through diet and fasting).

- Pulse = Targeted therapy to further weaken cancer cells (such as repurposed drugs like metformin, ivermectin, or hyperbaric oxygen therapy).

Seyfried's Conclusion: Cancer is highly vulnerable when both glucose and glutamine are restricted, combined with metabolic stressors.

Does Science Support This?

Studies show that ketogenic diets can slow tumour growth in mice and some human cases.

Human trials are ongoing, with promising case reports of ketogenic diets enhancing chemotherapy and improving survival rates.

Many oncologists remain sceptical, arguing that not all cancers are glucose-dependent and that more research is needed.

Seyfried's Conclusion: While not a "cure-all," a ketogenic diet is a powerful tool in a metabolic therapy strategy for fighting cancer.

Here's the link for the press and pulse strategy:

https://nutritionandmetabolism.biomedcentral.com/articles/10.1186/s12986-017-0178-2

Can Exercise Reduce Glutamine Availability for Cancer?

Yes, **exercise can help lower glutamine availability**, which may limit a key fuel source for cancer cells. Since **cancer thrives on both glucose and glutamine**, reducing either one can create a hostile environment for tumour growth.

1 Exercise Depletes Glutamine by Increasing Muscle Uptake

Skeletal muscle is the largest glutamine reservoir in the body.

During exercise, muscles consume large amounts of glutamine for energy, repair, and immune function.

This means less glutamine is available in the bloodstream for cancer cells to use.

Key Point: The more glutamine muscles take up, the less is left for tumours to feed on.

2 Exercise Enhances Mitochondrial Function in Healthy Cells

Cancer cells rely on glutamine fermentation (glutaminolysis) because of defective mitochondria.

Regular exercise improves mitochondrial efficiency in normal cells, making them less dependent on glutamine.

This means normal cells adapt, but cancer cells struggle under low-glutamine conditions.

Key Point: Exercise shifts energy metabolism away from glutamine dependence in healthy tissues.

3 High-Intensity Exercise Burns Through Glutamine Faster

Aerobic exercise (running, cycling, HIIT) increases glutamine demand in muscles.

Resistance training (weightlifting) stimulates muscle repair, which requires glutamine.

Since glutamine is constantly being used up, it cannot accumulate in high amounts for cancer cells.

Key Point: Frequent exercise keeps glutamine levels lower over time.

4 Exercise Enhances Immune Cell Consumption of Glutamine

Immune cells (T cells, macrophages) also use glutamine to function properly.

Exercise boosts immune activity, increasing their glutamine demand.

This diverts glutamine away from cancer cells, making tumours more vulnerable.

Key Point: More immune activation = less glutamine for cancer growth.

5 Exercise + Ketogenic Diet = Dual Glutamine Reduction Strategy

A ketogenic diet already lowers glucose, starving cancer of its primary fuel.

Exercise further reduces glutamine, hitting cancer from both sides.

This combination forces cancer cells into an energy crisis, potentially slowing tumour progression.

Key Point: Exercise + ketosis may be an effective metabolic strategy for fighting cancer.

What Type of Exercise Works Best?

Aerobic Exercise (Jogging, Cycling, Swimming) → Increases overall glutamine consumption.

Resistance Training (Weightlifting, Bodyweight Workouts) → Stimulates muscle growth, further pulling in glutamine.

HIIT (High-Intensity Interval Training) → Maximizes energy depletion, keeping glutamine levels low.

Best Approach: A mix of aerobic and resistance training, at least 3-5 times per week, to continuously lower glutamine levels.

Here's the link to read more about this:

https://pubmed.ncbi.nlm.nih.gov/32240949/

Associations Between Vitamin D Levels and Cancer

- **Increased Risk:** Some studies have found that low levels of vitamin D are associated with a higher risk of certain cancers, including breast, colorectal, and prostate cancers. For instance, research has suggested that higher vitamin D concentrations are linked to a threefold decrease in the risk of pancreatic cancer.

https://pmc.ncbi.nlm.nih.gov/articles/PMC3440651

- **Tumour Progression:** Vitamin D deficiency has been associated with tumour progression and metastasis in breast cancer, indicating that adequate levels may play a role in inhibiting cancer spread.

https://www.cancer.gov/news-events/cancer-currents-blog/2016/vitamin-d-metastasis

Vitamin D plays a crucial role in modulating the immune system, influencing both innate and adaptive immune responses.

Innate Immunity:

- **Antimicrobial Peptide Production:** Vitamin D stimulates the production of antimicrobial peptides, such as cathelicidin, which enhance the pathogen-fighting capabilities of immune cells.

https://pmc.ncbi.nlm.nih.gov/articles/PMC3738984

- **Monocyte and Dendritic Cell Regulation:** It influences the differentiation and activity of monocytes and dendritic cells, essential components of the innate immune system.

https://www.mdpi.com/1422-0067/23/17/9784

Adaptive Immunity:

- **T Cell Modulation:** Vitamin D affects T cell responses, promoting a balance that may reduce the risk of autoimmune reactions.

https://pubmed.ncbi.nlm.nih.gov/21527855/

- **B Cell Function:** It also influences B cell activity, impacting antibody production and contributing to immune regulation.

https://pmc.ncbi.nlm.nih.gov/articles/PMC3738984

Different People Produce Vitamin D at Different Rates

Not everyone synthesizes vitamin D efficiently from sunlight. Several factors can influence this, including:

Skin Color

Darker skin has more melanin, which acts as a natural sunscreen. This reduces the skin's ability to produce vitamin D.

People with darker skin tones may need 3 to 5 times more sun exposure than those with lighter skin.

Age

As people age, their skin produces less vitamin D because of reduced efficiency in converting UVB rays.

Older adults (especially over 60) are at higher risk of deficiency.

Genetics

Some people genetically have a lower ability to produce or metabolize vitamin D.

Variations in genes like CYP2R1 (involved in vitamin D activation) affect how efficiently someone can use vitamin D from sunlight.

Environmental & Lifestyle Factors Reduce Vitamin D Synthesis

Even if you spend time outdoors, several conditions may block or limit vitamin D production:

Sunscreen Use

SPF blocks UVB rays, reducing vitamin D synthesis by up to 95%.

While sun protection is important, brief exposure (10-30 minutes, depending on skin type) without sunscreen can help boost vitamin D.

Geographic Location (Latitude Matters!)

If you live farther from the equator, especially above 37° latitude, your winter sun is too weak for vitamin D production.

Countries like Canada, UK, Northern US, and parts of Europe experience vitamin D winter from November to March.

Time of Day

Vitamin D production is most effective between 10 AM and 3 PM.

If you're indoors during these peak hours, your vitamin D synthesis drops.

Air Pollution & Cloud Cover

High pollution levels block UVB rays.

Overcast skies reduce UV exposure by 50% or more.

Clothing & Cultural Norms

People who cover most of their skin (due to religious, cultural, or personal reasons) get little to no UVB exposure.

Even with Sunlight, Some People Don't Convert Vitamin D Well

Even if your skin makes vitamin D from sunlight, your body still needs to activate it—and this depends on liver and kidney function.

Liver or Kidney Disease

The liver converts vitamin D into 25(OH)D, the form measured in blood tests.

The kidneys convert it into the active form (1,25-dihydroxyvitamin D).

People with liver disease, kidney disease, or diabetes may struggle to activate vitamin D, leading to deficiency.

Obesity & Fat Absorption Issues

Vitamin D is fat-soluble, meaning it gets stored in body fat.

Obese individuals may trap vitamin D in fat stores, making less available for the body to use.

People with gut issues (Crohn's, celiac disease, IBS, gastric bypass) may have trouble absorbing dietary vitamin D.

Should You Supplement?

Because so many factors affect vitamin D levels, supplementation may be necessary for some people. General guidelines:

Mild Deficiency: 1,000–2,000 IU/day

Moderate Deficiency: 5,000 IU/day

Severe Deficiency: 10,000 IU/day (under medical supervision)

- Best Form?

Vitamin D3 (cholecalciferol) is preferred over D2 (ergocalciferol) because it's more effective.

- Pair with Vitamin K2?

Helps direct calcium to bones instead of arteries, reducing calcification risks.

- Take with Fat?

Since vitamin D is fat-soluble, taking it with a fatty meal increases absorption.

Sun exposure isn't always enough—genetics, skin color, location, lifestyle, and health conditions all affect vitamin D production.

Many people may need supplements, especially those who live in cold climates, have darker skin, are older, or have metabolic issues.

Regular blood tests (25(OH)D) can confirm if you need supplementation.

Why Curcumin for Cancer?

Curcumin, the active compound in **turmeric**, has been widely studied for its **anti-cancer properties**. Research suggests that it can **inhibit cancer cell growth, reduce inflammation, and even make cancer cells more vulnerable to treatment**.

Curcumin Disrupts Cancer Cell Growth & Proliferation

Cancer cells divide uncontrollably due to faulty signaling pathways.

Curcumin blocks multiple cancer-promoting pathways (like NF-κB, STAT3, and mTOR), slowing tumour growth.

It also interferes with cancer stem cells, which are responsible for metastasis and recurrence.

Key Study: Curcumin was shown to inhibit tumour growth in multiple cancer types, including breast, colon, prostate, and lung cancers.

https://pubmed.ncbi.nlm.nih.gov/21872638/

Curcumin Induces Apoptosis (Forcing Cancer Cells to Self-Destruct)

Healthy cells die naturally through a process called apoptosis, but cancer cells avoid this.

Curcumin reactivates apoptosis in cancer cells by regulating p53, Bax, and caspases, making it harder for tumours to survive.

Key Study: Curcumin induced apoptosis in lung cancer cells, leading to a reduction in tumour size.

https://pmc.ncbi.nlm.nih.gov/articles/PMC2644749/

Curcumin Starves Cancer by Cutting Off Blood Supply (Anti-Angiogenesis)

Tumours grow by forming new blood vessels (angiogenesis) to supply oxygen and nutrients.

Curcumin blocks VEGF (Vascular Endothelial Growth Factor), preventing tumours from forming new blood vessels.

Key Study: A study in colorectal cancer found that curcumin reduced blood vessel formation, slowing tumor progression.

https://pmc.ncbi.nlm.nih.gov/articles/PMC4637299/

Check out this link to know more:

https://pmc.ncbi.nlm.nih.gov/articles/PMC2758121/

Chapter 8: A Final Thank You

To everyone who has purchased this book—thank you from the bottom of my heart.

This isn't just a story about my dad's fight against cancer. It's a testament to resilience, hope, and the power of knowledge. Every bit of research, every change in strategy, every decision we made was driven by one goal: to give him a fighting chance.

The funds from this book are not for profit—they go directly toward improving his quality of life, whether it's for better nutrition, supplements, treatments, or simply making his days more comfortable.

By reading this, you are part of his journey. You are helping us continue the fight.

If this book has given you even one useful insight, one new way to see cancer differently, or one spark of hope, then sharing our story has been worth it.

Thank you for being here. Thank you for caring.

� With gratitude,

M.

Don't miss out!

Visit the website below and you can sign up to receive emails whenever M. publishes a new book. There's no charge and no obligation.

https://books2read.com/r/B-A-HMZJD-KBVZF

BOOKS 2 READ

Connecting independent readers to independent writers.

www.ingramcontent.com/pod-product-compliance
Lightning Source LLC
LaVergne TN
LVHW101617210926
848480LV00009B/750
* 9 7 9 8 2 3 0 1 7 4 0 7 3 *